The Complete Alkaline Cookbook

Simple and Tasty

Alkaline Recipes for a Healthy

Lifestyle

Sam Carter

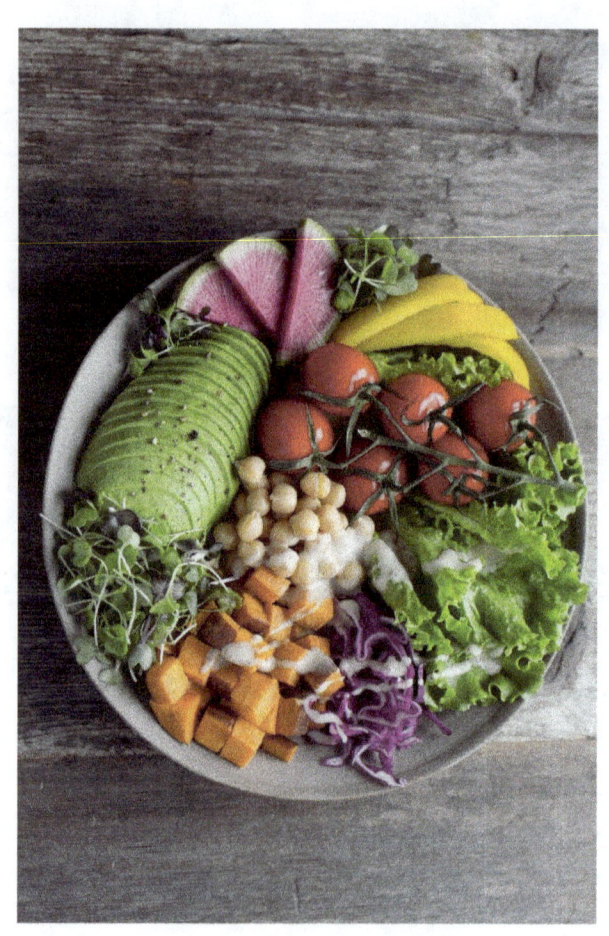

© **Copyright 2021 - All rights reserved.**

The content contained within this book may not be reproduced, duplicated or transmitted without direct written permission from the author or the publisher.

Under no circumstances will any blame or legal responsibility be held against the publisher, or author, for any damages, reparation, or monetary loss due to the information contained within this book. Either directly or indirectly.

Legal Notice:

This book is copyright protected. This book is only for personal use. You cannot amend, distribute, sell, use, quote or paraphrase any part, or the content within this book, without the consent of the author or publisher.

Disclaimer Notice:

Please note the information contained within this document is for educational and entertainment purposes only. All effort has been executed to present accurate, up to date, and reliable, complete information. No warranties of any kind are declared or implied. Readers acknowledge that the author is not engaging in the rendering of legal, financial, medical or professional advice. The content within this book has been derived from various sources. Please consult a licensed professional before attempting any techniques outlined in this book.

By reading this document, the reader agrees that under no circumstances is the author responsible for any losses, direct or indirect, which are incurred as a result of the use of information contained within this document, including, but not limited to, — errors, omissions, or inaccuracies.

Table of Contents

Zesty Green Chips 7
Mediterranean Spread 9
Summer Fruit Soup 11
Carrot Tahini Slaw 13
Veggie Chips 15
Spiced Middle Eastern Dip 17
Detox Soup 20
Vegetarian Paté 22
Sage & Butternut Squash Soup 24
Chilled Tomato Soup 26
Sweet & Sour Cabbage 29
Vegetable & Lentil Soup 31
Roasted Red Pepper Dip 34
Ghee & Maple Roasted Carrots 36
Edamame Salad 38
Smokey Caesar Salad 39
Baked Sweet Potato Fries with Spicy BBQ Sauce 41
Citrus & Jicama Salad 44
Green Cabbage Slaw 46
Spicy Mix with Tortilla Chips 48
Creamy Broccoli Soup 50
Chilled Coconut Soup 52
Root Vegetable Soup 54
Squash Dip with Cucumber Slices 56
Creamy Two Bean Salad 58

Fruit Porridge	62
Morning Sweet Bread	64
Banana Breakfast Pudding	66
Italian Breakfast Hash	68
Papaya Breakfast Boat	70
AM Quinoa Cookies	72
Savory Breakfast Bowl	74
Almond Butter & Jelly Overnight Oats	76
Broccoli & Sprouts Savory Oats	78
Fruit & Millet Breakfast	80
Avocado Breakfast Soup	83
Greek Zucchini Cups	86
Endive & Watercress Boats	88
Chickpea Avocado Cups	90
Spicy Cocoa-Coco Truffles	92
Asian Cucumber Slaw	95
Broiled Grapefruit	96
Coconut Curry Soup	97
Chilled Avocado Cilantro Soup	100
Cooling Cucumber Slice Snack	102
Spicy Tortilla Soup	104
Raw Green Gazpacho	106

Zesty Green Chips

Servings: 2

Total Time: 5 minutes plus 2 hours chill time

Ingredients

- 1 bunch kale, stems removed and torn into large pieces
- 1 tablespoon olive oil
- 1 teaspoon Himalayan salt
- 1 teaspoon black pepper, crushed
- 1 teaspoon cayenne pepper
- 1 teaspoon chili powder
- 2 tablespoons nutritional yeast

Directions

1. Preheat oven to 300°F/150°C and line 2 baking trays with parchment paper.

2. Place kale in a large bowl and pour olive oil on top. Massage kale gently until fully coated.

3. In a small bowl combine salt, pepper, cayenne, chili powder and nutritional yeast. Sprinkle mixture over the kale and make sure every piece is covered with the spice mixture.

4. Lay kale pieces on the baking tray making sure they are in an even layer. Bake 10 minutes, flip pieces over and bake an additional 10 minutes.

5. Remove from oven and let cool.

Mediterranean Spread

Servings: 2

Total Time: 5 minutes plus 2 hours chill time

Ingredients

- ¼ cup pitted black olives
- ¼ cup pitted green olives
- ¼ cup sundried tomatoes, chopped
- 1 garlic clove, minced
- 1 teaspoon Dijon mustard
- 1 teaspoon fresh thyme leaves, chopped
- 1 teaspoon fresh oregano, chopped
- 2 tablespoons chopped parsley
- ½ lemon, juiced
- 3 tablespoons olive oil
- 1 small Belgian endive, leaves cleaned and trimmed
- Spelt crackers (optional)

Directions

1. In a food processor combine the black and green olives, tomatoes, garlic, mustard, thyme, oregano and parsley. Scrape down sides and add in lemon juice. Slowly, with the food processor running, drizzle in olive oil.

2. Serve with endive leaves or spelt crackers.

Summer Fruit Soup

Servings: 2

Total Time: 5 minutes plus 1 hour chill time

Ingredients

- 1 cup cantaloupe, cubed
- 1 cup watermelon, cubed
- 1 cup honeydew, cubed
- 2 tablespoons lime juice
- 1 cup unsweetened coconut milk
- ½ cup water
- 1 tablespoon raw honey
- ⅛ teaspoon Himalayan salt
- 1 tablespoon mint leaves, chopped
- 4 raspberries

Directions

1. In a food processor combine the cantaloupe, watermelon, honeydew, lime juice, coconut milk, water, honey and salt.

2. Chill 1 hour in the fridge. Garnish with mint and raspberries before serving.

Carrot Tahini Slaw

Servings: 2

Total Time: 15 minutes

Ingredients

- 1 ½ cups carrots, shredded
- 1 cup red cabbage, shredded
- 1 tablespoon green onions, sliced
- 2 tablespoons raisins
- 3 tablespoons tahini paste
- 1 teaspoon ginger, grated
- 2 teaspoons warm water
- 1 teaspoon lemon juice
- 1 teaspoon raw honey
- ¼ teaspoon Himalayan salt

Directions

1. In a small bowl whisk together the tahini, ginger, water, lemon juice, honey and salt until smooth. If mixture is too thick, thin out with more water.

2. Mix together the carrots, cabbage, raisins and green onions in a large bowl. Drizzle tahini sauce over vegetables and toss to combine. Let sit for 10 minutes before serving.

Veggie Chips

Servings: 2

Total Time: 15 minutes

Ingredients

- 1 large zucchini, sliced thin
- 1 small beet, peeled and sliced thin
- 1 tablespoon olive oil
- ¼ teaspoon Himalayan salt
- 1 teaspoon garlic powder

Directions

1. Place zucchini and beet slices on paper towel or tea towel and let sit for 10 minutes to draw out any moisture. Blot slices dry with a fresh towel.

2. Preheat oven to 200°F/95°C and line a baking tray with parchment paper.

3. Place vegetable slices on baking tray in single layer. Brush each side lightly with olive oil and sprinkle with salt and garlic powder.

4. Bake in the oven for 60 minutes or until crispy. Let cool completely.

Spiced Middle Eastern Dip

Servings: 2

Total Time: 15 minutes

Ingredients

- 1 eggplant, sliced into rounds
- ½ teaspoon Himalayan salt
- 1 tablespoon olive oil
- ½ teaspoon olive oil (extra)
- 2 garlic cloves, peeled and grated
- 1 shallot, sliced
- ¼ teaspoon cumin
- ¼ teaspoon red chili flakes
- ⅛ teaspoon black pepper, crushed
- ½ cup parsley, chopped
- 1 tablespoon tahini
- 1 ½ tablespoons lemon juice or more to taste
- ¼ teaspoon Himalayan salt
- 1 cucumber, sliced

Directions

1. Place eggplant slices on paper or tea towel and sprinkle with ¼ teaspoon salt. Let sit 10 minutes to draw out water. Rinse eggplant and blot dry.

2. Place eggplant slices on a baking tray lined with parchment paper, drizzle with 1 tablespoon olive oil and ¼ teaspoon salt. Roast eggplant in the oven's broiler on high for 5 - 8 minutes or until lightly browned and soft. Remove from oven and peel away the skin.

3. In a food processor, add the eggplant flesh, garlic, shallot, cumin, chili flakes parsley, tahini, lemon juice, remaining ¼ teaspoon salt. Process until well combined.

4. While the food processor is running, drizzle in remaining olive oil. Serve with sliced cucumber.

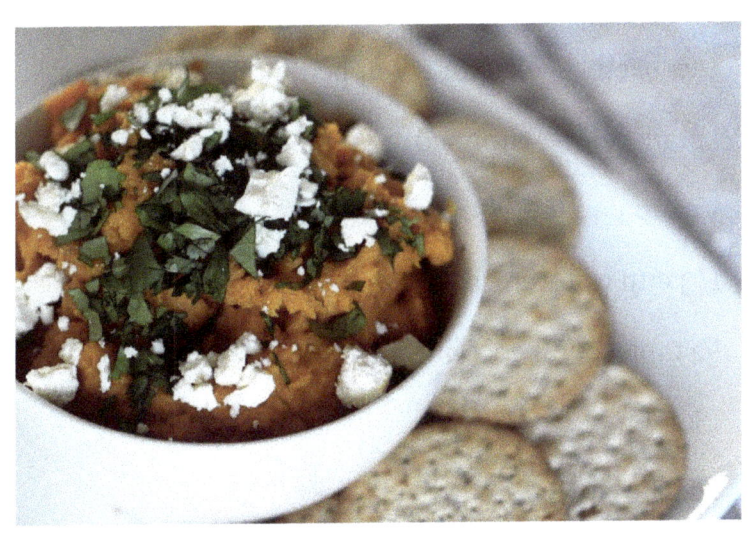

Detox Soup

Servings: 2

Total Time: 15 minutes

Ingredients

- 1 ½ beets, peeled and chopped into 1 inch pieces
- 1 stalk celery, chopped
- ½ cup parsley, chopped
- 1/3 cup watercress
- ½ tablespoon coconut oil
- 1 lemon, juiced
- 1 garlic clove, minced
- 2 cups water
- 2 tablespoons apple cider vinegar
- ⅛ teaspoon cayenne pepper

Directions

1. In a medium saucepan over medium heat, add coconut oil, celery, beets, garlic and lemon juice. Cook 8 minutes until soft.

2. Add water, vinegar and cayenne and bring to a boil.

3. Reduce heat and stir in parsley and watercress. Cook 1 minutes and turn heat off before serving.

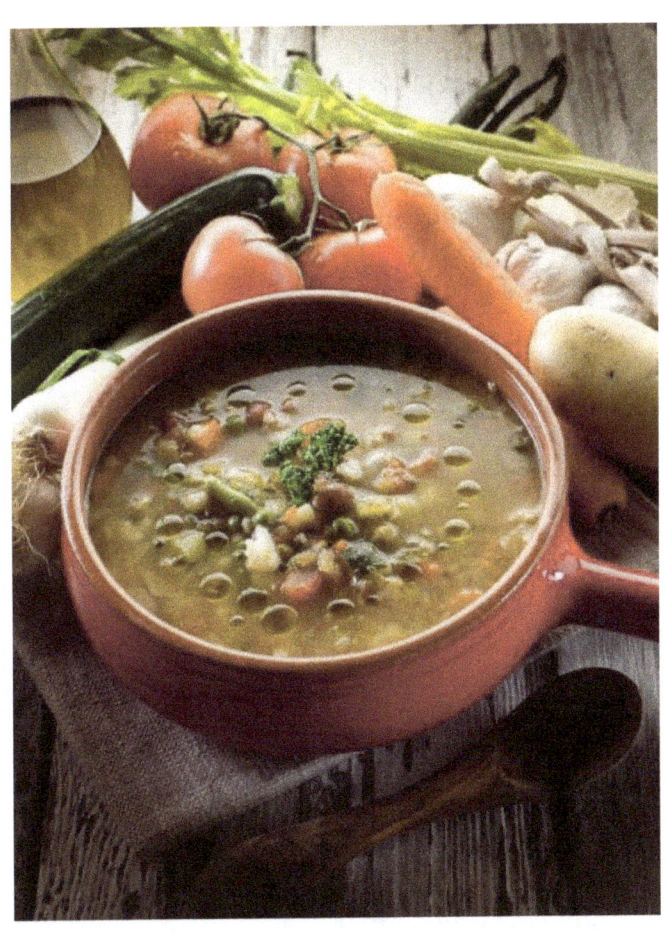

Vegetarian Paté

Servings: 2

Total Time: 20 minutes

Ingredients

- 1 cup green lentils, cooked
- 1 tablespoon olive oil
- ½ cup button mushrooms, sliced
- ½ onion, chopped
- 1 garlic clove, minced
- 2 tablespoons walnuts, toasted
- 1 ½ tablespoons tamari
- ½ cup parsley, chopped
- 1 tablespoon fresh sage, chopped
- ¼ teaspoon black pepper, crushed
- ½ teaspoon Himalayan salt
- 1 teaspoon Dijon mustard
- 1 teaspoon cayenne pepper
- ¼ cup water

- 1 cucumber sliced

Directions

1. In a medium saucepan over medium-low heat, add olive oil, onions, mushrooms, and garlic. Cook 8 minutes until soft.

2. In a food processor combine the mushroom onion mixture with the cooked green lentils, walnuts, tamari, parsley, sage, pepper, salt, mustard, cayenne pepper and water. Combine until smooth, adding more water if needed. Transfer to a bowl and refrigerate until ready to serve.

3. Serve with cucumber slices

Sage & Butternut Squash Soup

Servings: 2

Total Time: 25 minutes

Ingredients

- 3 tablespoons olive oil
- 2 shallots, sliced
- 1 garlic clove, minced
- 1 medium butternut squash, peeled and cubed
- 5 fresh sage leaves
- 3 cups vegetable broth
- 1 tablespoon maple syrup
- 1 teaspoon Himalayan salt
- 1 teaspoon black pepper, crushed
- ¼ teaspoon nutmeg
- ¼ cup unsweetened almond milk

Directions

1. In a medium saucepan over medium-low heat, add 2 tablespoons of olive oil, shallot and garlic and cook 5 minutes until soft. Add in butternut squash, 3 sage leaves, broth, maple syrup, salt, pepper and nutmeg.

2. Bring mixture to a boil, reduce heat and simmer 20 minutes or until squash is soft.

3. When mixture is cooled, add to blender and blend until smooth. Add back to saucepan and bring to a simmer. Pour in almond milk and cook 3 minutes.

4. In a small saucepan over low heat, add 1 tablespoon of oil. When oil is warm, add the 2 unused sage leaves and cook 4 minutes being sure not to burn. Remove sage leaves and set aside.

5. Pour soup into serving bowls and top with frizzled sage leaves.

Chilled Tomato Soup

Servings: 2

Total Time: 10 minutes plus 2 hours chill time

Ingredients

- 3 tomatoes, peeled
- ½ large green bell pepper, finely chopped
- 1 ½ tablespoons apple cider vinegar
- 1 ½ tablespoons lemon juice
- 1 ½ cucumber, peeled, seeded and finely diced
- 2 shallots, sliced
- 1 jalapeno, seeded and diced
- 1 teaspoon cumin
- 1 teaspoon tamari
- 1 tablespoon olive oil
- 1 ½ tablespoons fresh parsley, chopped
- 1 tablespoon
- 1 teaspoon sugar free hot sauce

Directions

1. Place all ingredients in a blend and combine until full mixed (mixture will not be entirely smooth). If a thinner soup is desired, add 1 tablespoon of water at a time until desired consistency is achieved.

2. Chill in the fridge for 2 hours before serving.

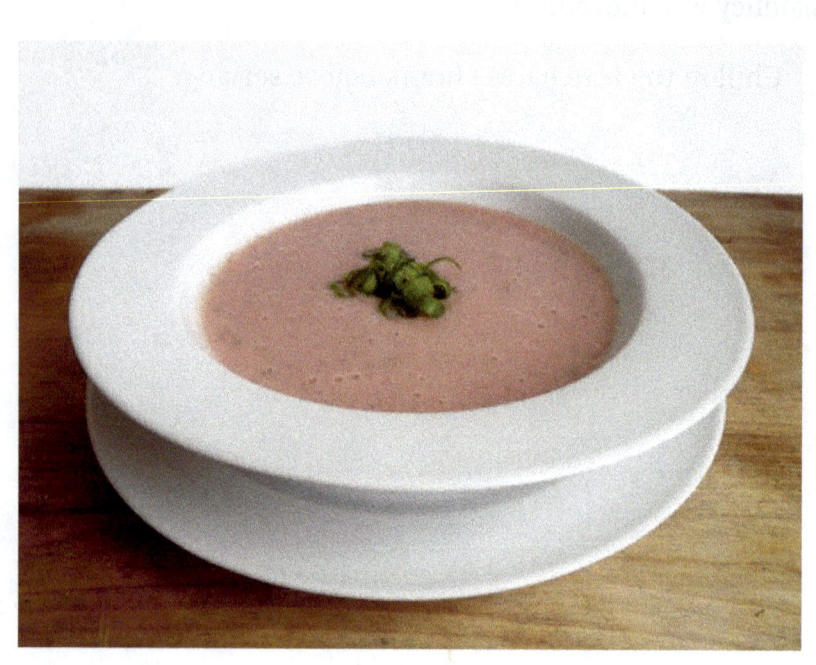

Sweet & Sour Cabbage

Servings: 2

Total Time: 45 minutes

Ingredients

- 1 teaspoon ghee
- 1 teaspoon olive oil
- 1 shallot, thinly sliced
- ½ green cabbage, shredded
- ½ red cabbage, shredded
- 2 tablespoons raw honey
- ½ cup apple cider vinegar
- 1/3 cup water
- 1 teaspoon Himalayan salt
- 1 teaspoon black pepper, crushed
- ½ teaspoon nutmeg
- 1 tablespoon caraway seeds

Directions

1. In a large pot, heat ghee and olive oil over medium heat and add the shallot, green and red cabbage. Cook for 10 minutes or until softened and coated with the oil and ghee.

2. Add honey, vinegar, water, salt, pepper and nutmeg. Cook another 5 minutes then reduce heat to low and simmer for 30 minutes or until cabbage is soft.

3. Stir in caraway seeds and serve warm.

Vegetable & Lentil Soup

Servings: 2

Total Time: 1 hour

Ingredients

- ½ tablespoon olive oil
- 1 garlic clove, minced
- ¼ cup carrots, diced
- ¼ cup celery, diced
- ¼ cup yellow onion, diced
- 1 small leek, white part sliced into half-moons and cleaned well
- ½ cup brown lentils, washed and drained
- 1 teaspoon dried rosemary
- 1 teaspoon dried thyme
- 2 cups water
- 1 tablespoon tomato paste
- 1 tablespoon apple cider vinegar
- 1 teaspoon Himalayan salt

- 1 teaspoon black pepper, crushed
- Handful spinach leaves

Directions

1. In a large pot, olive oil and add garlic, onion, carrot, celery and onion. After 5 minutes add the leeks and cook an additional 10 minutes.

2. Add the lentils, rosemary, thyme, water, tomato paste and vinegar. Cook, uncovered, for 45 minutes or until lentils are tender. Stir in spinach leaves and season with salt and pepper before serving.

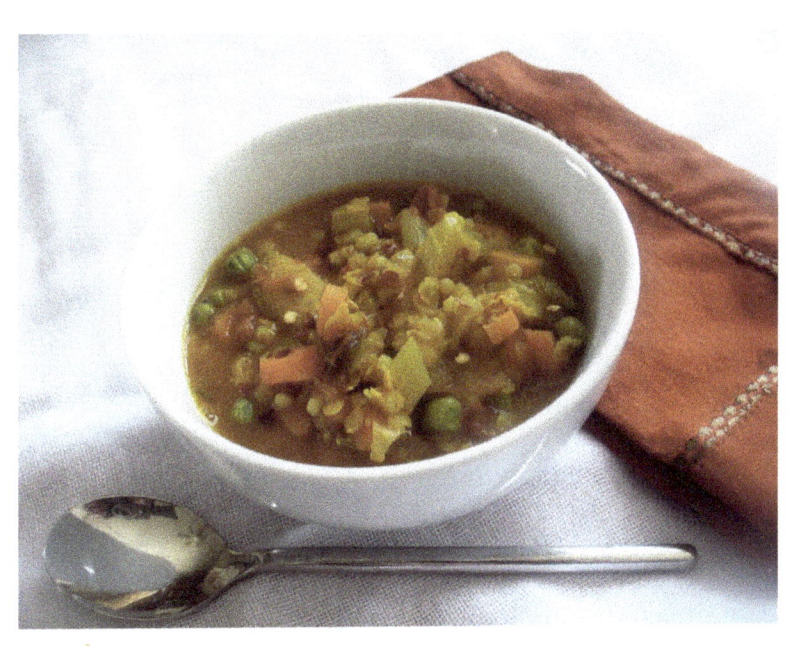

Roasted Red Pepper Dip

Servings: 2

Total Time: 5 minutes

Ingredients

- 2 whole roasted peppers
- ¾ cup walnuts, toasted
- ½ cup green onions, sliced
- 2 garlic cloves
- ½ teaspoon Himalayan salt
- 1 tablespoon lemon juice
- 2 teaspoons raw honey
- 1 teaspoon ground cumin
- 1 teaspoon red chili flakes
- ½ teaspoon cayenne pepper
- ½ teaspoon red pepper flakes
- 3 tablespoons almond meal
- 4 tablespoons olive oil

Directions

1. In a blender or food processor, combine all ingredients except leave a remaining 2 tablespoons of the olive oil.

2. Blend until smooth and transfer to serving bowl. Stir in the remaining 2 tablespoons of olive oil.

Ghee & Maple Roasted Carrots

Servings: 2

Total Time: 35 minutes

Ingredients

- 3 large carrots, washed and cut into 1 inch pieces
- 1 tablespoon ghee, melted
- 1 tablespoon maple syrup
- 1 teaspoon lemon zest
- 1 teaspoon Himalayan salt
- ¼ teaspoon black pepper, crushed
- 1 tablespoon sesame seeds, toasted

Directions

1. Preheat oven to 400°F/205°C.

2. In a small bowl, whisk together the ghee, maple syrup, lemon zest, salt and pepper.

3. Place carrots in a shallow baking dish and coat with ghee and maple mixture. Roast 25 minutes, turning once halfway through.

4. Remove carrots from oven and sprinkle the sesame seeds.

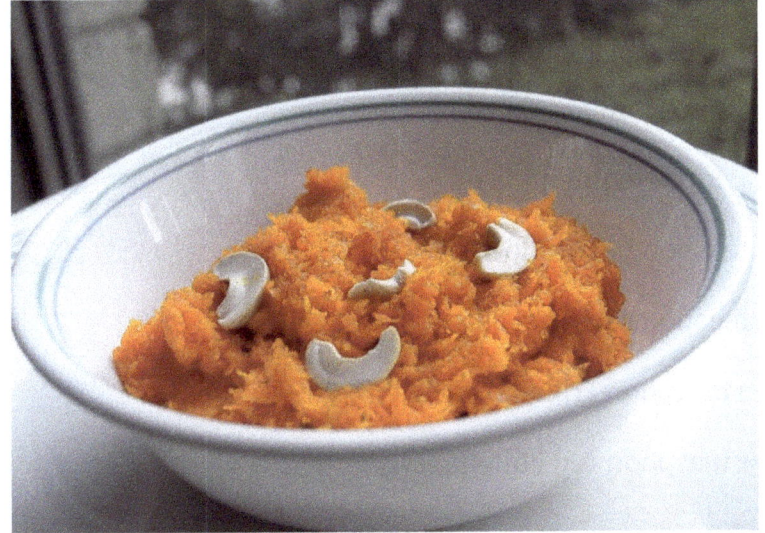

Edamame Salad

Servings: 2

Total Time: 20 minutes

Ingredients

- 1 cup edamame, shelled, cooked and cooled
- 2 tablespoons green onions, sliced
- 1 cup cucumber, diced
- ¼ cup red onion, diced
- 1 teaspoon avocado oil
- 1 teaspoon sesame oil
- ½ teaspoon Himalayan salt
- ¼ teaspoon red chili flakes

Directions

1. Toss all ingredients in a medium bowl and make sure it is all well coated.
2. Chill in the fridge for 15 minutes before serving.

Smokey Caesar Salad

Servings: 2

Total Time: 15 minutes

Ingredients

- 1 large bunch kale, stems removes and thinly sliced
- 1 cup pumpkin seeds
- 5 cherry tomatoes, halved
- ½ cucumber, diced
- 1/3 cup almonds
- ⅛ teaspoon chipotle powder
- ½ teaspoon smoked paprika
- 2 garlic cloves
- 1 tablespoon nutritional yeast
- 1 ¼ cup filtered water
- 1 teaspoon honey
- ½ teaspoon Himalayan salt

Directions

1. In a blender combine the almonds, chipotle powder, smoked paprika, garlic, nutritional yeast, water, honey and salt.

2. Place kale, pumpkin seeds, cherry tomatoes and cucumber in a large bowl and cover with dressing mix from the blender.

3. Toss well to ensure all the leaves are coated and let sit a few minutes before serving.

Baked Sweet Potato Fries with Spicy BBQ Sauce

Servings: 2

Total Time: 35 minutes

Ingredients

- 1 large sweet potato, cut into large julienne sticks
- 1 tablespoon avocado oil
- ½ teaspoon Himalayan salt
- ½ teaspoon garlic powder

Spicy BBQ Sauce

- 2 tablespoons tomato paste
- 1 tablespoon water
- 1 tablespoon maple syrup
- 1 tablespoon coconut aminos
- 1 teaspoon tamari
- 1 teaspoon smoked paprika
- 1 teaspoon chili powder
- ½ teaspoon cayenne pepper

Directions

1. Make Spicy BBQ Sauce by combining all the Spicy BBQ Sauce ingredients in a blender.

2. Preheat oven to 400°F/205°C. In a large bowl, toss sweet potato with oil, salt and garlic powder.

3. Place sweet potato on one layer of parchment paper lined on a baking tray. Bake 20 minutes, flipping halfway through.

4. Serve sweet potato fries with the Spicy BBQ Sauce.

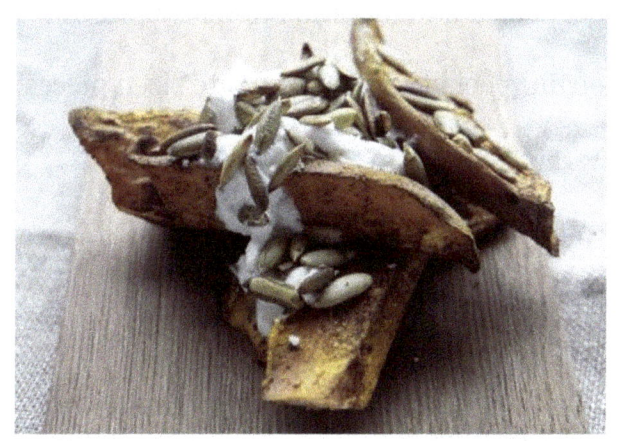

Citrus & Jicama Salad

Servings: 2

Total Time: 35 minutes

Ingredients

- 1 orange, peeled and cut into bite-sized pieces
- 1 grapefruit, peeled and cut into bite sized pieces
- 1 jicama, shredded
- 3 cups spinach
- 3 tablespoons green onions, thinly sliced
- ½ head radicchio, thinly sliced
- 2 tablespoons olive oil
- 2 tablespoons orange juice
- 1 tablespoon lemon juice
- 1 teaspoon lemon zest
- ¼ teaspoon Himalayan salt
- ⅛ teaspoon ground cloves
- ⅛ teaspoon black pepper, crushed

Directions

1. In a large bowl, combine orange pieces, grapefruit pieces, shredded jicama, spinach, green onions and radicchio.

2. Whisk together the olive oil, orange juice, lemon juice, lemon zest, salt, ground cloves and black pepper in a small bowl to form the dressing.

3. Pour dressing over the citrus and jicama salad and serve.

Green Cabbage Slaw

Servings: 2

Total Time: 15 minutes

Ingredients

- 1 avocado
- 3 tablespoons olive oil
- 1 lemon, juiced
- 1 teaspoon apple cider vinegar
- ¼ teaspoon Himalayan salt
- ½ cup green cabbage, thinly shredded
- 2 carrots, shredded
- 2 shallots, thinly sliced
- 3 tablespoons cilantro, finely chopped
- 1 tablespoon green onions, thinly sliced
- 1 tablespoon raisins

Directions

1. Place avocado, olive oil, lemon juice, vinegar and salt in a blender and combine until smooth.

2. In a large bowl combine the avocado mixture, cabbage, carrots, shallots, cilantro, green onion and raisins.

3. Chill 10 minutes before serving.

Spicy Mix with Tortilla Chips

Servings: 2

Total Time: 5 minutes plus 30 minutes chill time

Ingredients

- 3 tomatoes, finely diced
- 1 green bell pepper, seeded and finely diced
- 2 green onions, thinly sliced
- 2 garlic cloves, grated
- 1 jalapeno, seeded and finely diced
- 2 tablespoons cilantro, finely chopped
- ½ teaspoon Himalayan salt
- ½ teaspoon cayenne pepper
- ¼ teaspoon red chili flakes
- 1 lime, juiced
- 1 tablespoon olive oil
- 24 sprouted corn tortilla chips

Directions

1. In a medium bowl combine all the ingredients except the tortilla chips. Place half of the mixture in a blender or food processor and pulse 10 times.

2. Add blended mix back to the bowl with the rest of ingredients and stir to combine.

3. Chill at least 30 minutes before serving with tortilla chips.

Creamy Broccoli Soup

Servings: 2

Total Time: 30 minutes

Ingredients

- 1 small head broccoli, cut into florets
- 1 small avocado
- 1 large shallot, diced
- 1 tablespoon coconut oil
- 1 cup vegetable broth
- ½ cup coconut milk
- 1 teaspoon Himalayan salt
- ½ teaspoon nutmeg
- ½ teaspoon black pepper, crushed

Directions

1. In a medium saucepan, heat coconut oil over medium high heat. Add shallot and broccoli and cook 10 minutes. Pour in vegetable broth and coconut milk.

2. Bring to a simmer and cook 15 minutes. Let cool and add to blender or food processor along with the avocado and blend until smooth.

3. Add back to saucepan and bring to a simmer. Stir in salt, nutmeg and black pepper.

Chilled Coconut Soup

Servings: 2

Total Time: 5 minutes plus 3 hours chill time

Ingredients

- 1 small head cauliflower, steamed or roasted
- 1 cup unsweetened coconut milk
- 1 cup water
- 2 tablespoons lime juice
- 2 tablespoons coconut oil
- 1 tablespoon cream of coconut
- 2 teaspoons cilantro, chopped

Directions

1. Add cauliflower, coconut milk, water, lime juice, coconut oil and cream of coconut in a food processor. Blend until smooth, adding more water if it is too thick.

2. Transfer to a large bowl and chill 2-3 hours. Garnish with cilantro before serving.

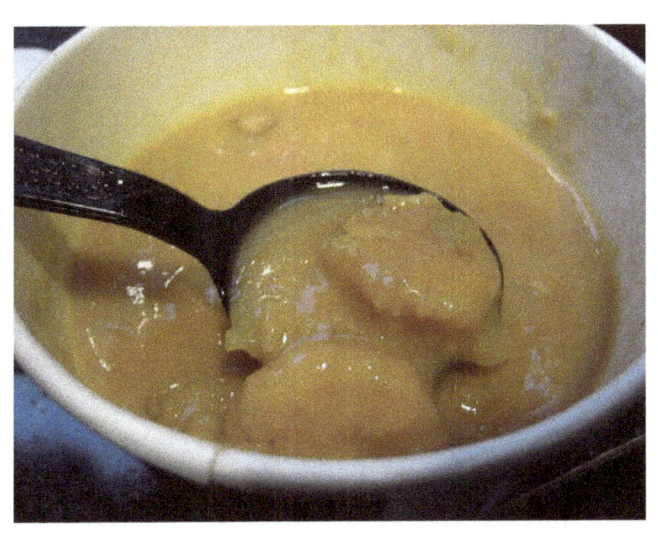

Root Vegetable Soup

Servings: 2

Total Time: 35 minutes

Ingredients

- 2 tablespoons coconut oil
- 2 medium shallots, sliced
- 1 inch piece ginger, peeled and sliced
- 4 carrots, chopped
- 1 sweet potato, peeled and chopped
- 2 parsnips, chopped
- 3 cups vegetable stock
- 1 teaspoon Himalayan salt
- 1 teaspoon black pepper, crushed
- ¼ teaspoon cinnamon
- ⅛ teaspoon nutmeg

Directions

1. Heat oil over medium heat in a medium saucepan. Add shallots and ginger and cook 5 minutes. Add carrots, sweet potato and parsnips. Cook another 10 minutes, stirring frequently.

2. In the saucepan, add the vegetable stock and bring to a boil. Reduce heat and simmer for 20 minutes or until vegetables are soft.

3. Let mixture cool before adding to a blender and mixing until smooth. If using an immersion blender, skip cooling the mixture.

4. Transfer back to saucepan and bring to a simmer over low heat. Stir in salt, pepper, cinnamon and nutmeg.

Squash Dip with Cucumber Slices

Servings: 2

Total Time: 5 minutes

Ingredients

- 1 cup pumpkin puree
- 1 avocado, pitted and flesh removed
- ½ red bell pepper, chopped
- 2 green onions, chopped
- 1 teaspoon cumin
- 1 teaspoon coriander
- 1 teaspoon ground cardamom
- ½ teaspoon turmeric
- ½ teaspoon cinnamon
- 1 tablespoon lemon juice
- 1 teaspoon Himalayan salt
- 1 teaspoon black pepper, crushed
- 1/3 cup water
- 1 cucumber, sliced

Directions

1. Add all the ingredients except the cucumber to a high speed blender and combine until smooth to create the dip.

2. Serve with cucumber slices.

Creamy Two Bean Salad

Servings: 2

Total Time: 10 minutes

Ingredients

- 1 cup white beans
- 1 cup celery, chopped
- ½ cup fresh green beans, chopped into 1 inch pieces
- ½ cup chopped organic red onion, or green onion
- 1 cup watercress
- 1 apple, chopped

Dressing

- 2 inch piece of fresh ginger peeled and sliced thin across the grain
- 2 tablespoons coconut oil
- 1 lime, juiced
- 1 tablespoon raw honey
- 1 teaspoon Himalayan salt
- 1 cup coconut milk

- ½ cup coconut cream
- 1 teaspoon, black pepper

Directions

1. Combine white beans, celery, green beans, onion, watercress and apple in a large bowl.

2. In a blender combine Dressing ingredients until smooth.

3. Pour Dressing over bean mixture and toss to coat.

4. Serve immediately.

Chilled Beet Soup

Servings: 2

Total Time: 30 minutes

Ingredients

- 1 tablespoon coconut oil
- 1/3 cup yellow onion, diced
- 1 cup beets, peeled and chopped
- 1/3 cup carrots, shredded
- 1 cup red cabbage, shredded
- 2 cups vegetable broth
- 1 teaspoon Himalayan salt
- 1 teaspoon black pepper, crushed
- 1 tablespoon fresh dill, chopped
- ½ cup unsweetened coconut milk

Directions

1. In a large saucepan over medium heat, add the coconut oil, onion, beets and carrots. Cook 10 minutes before adding the cabbage.

2. Cook an additional 5 minutes and add vegetable broth, salt, pepper and dill. Reduce heat to low and simmer for 15 minutes.

3. Using an immersion blender, blend mixture until smooth. Stir in coconut milk, transfer to a bowl and allow to sit for 5 minutes before serving.

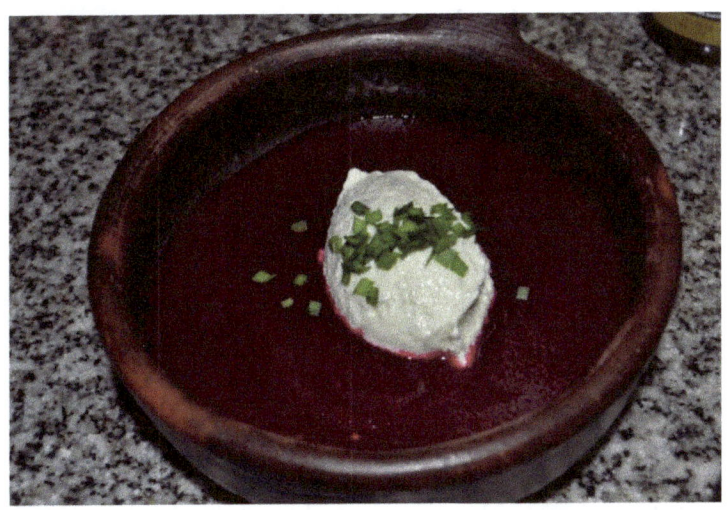

Fruit Porridge

Servings: 2

Total Time: 25 minutes

Ingredients

- ½ cup whole buckwheat
- ½ cup water
- ½ cup unsweetened almond milk
- 1 tablespoon dried apricot, diced
- 2 tablespoons raisins
- 1 cinnamon stick
- ¼ teaspoon nutmeg
- ¼ teaspoon vanilla extract
- 1 teaspoon ground cardamom
- 1 tablespoon pomegranate seeds
- 1 tablespoon walnuts, toasted and crushed

Directions

1. In a medium saucepan, add buckwheat, water, almond milk, apricot, raisins, cinnamon, nutmeg, vanilla and cardamom. Bring to a boil and then allow to simmer, stir frequently for 20 minutes or until liquid is absorbed.

2. Remove from heat, remove cinnamon stick and garnish with pomegranate seeds and walnuts before serving.

Morning Sweet Bread

Servings: 2

Total Time: 30 minutes

Ingredients

- 1 tablespoon flaxseed, ground
- 3 tablespoons water
- 1 ½ cups almond meal
- 2 tablespoons coconut flour
- 1 teaspoon Himalayan salt
- 2 teaspoon cinnamon
- 1 teaspoon vanilla extract
- 1 teaspoon raw honey
- 1 tablespoon olive oil
- 2 tablespoons raisins
- 1 tablespoon cashew butter, melted
- 1 pear, cored and sliced

Directions

1. Preheat oven to 350°F/180°C and line bottom of a small glass baking dish with parchment paper.

2. In a small bowl, mix together the flaxseeds and 3 tablespoons water to from the flaxseeds gel. Set aside and let sit 10 minutes until it forms a gel.

3. In a large bowl, combine the almond meal, coconut flour, salt, cinnamon, vanilla, honey, flaxseeds gel, olive oil and raisins.

4. Place dough in the baking dish and press into an even layer. Bake in the oven for 15 minutes.

5. Remove and let cool. Top with cashew butter and pear slices before serving.

Banana Breakfast Pudding

Servings: 1

Total Time: 5 minutes plus 8 hours chill time

Ingredients

- 1 cup coconut milk
- 1 tablespoon raw honey
- ½ teaspoon vanilla extract
- ¼ teaspoon cinnamon
- ¼ teaspoon nutmeg
- ⅛ teaspoon Himalayan salt
- 2 tablespoons chia seeds
- 1 banana, sliced
- 1 tablespoon walnuts, toasted and crushed
- 1 tablespoon cacao nibs

Directions

1. In a small bowl or jar with a cover, place coconut milk, honey, vanilla, cinnamon, nutmeg, salt and chia seeds.

2. Let sit in the fridge, covered, overnight.

3. In the morning, top with banana, walnuts and cacao nibs before serving.

Italian Breakfast Hash

Servings: 2

Total Time: 35 minutes

Ingredients

- 2 sweet potatoes, peeled and cubed into ½ inch pieces
- 2 tablespoons olive oil
- ½ red onion, chopped
- ½ red bell pepper, halved and sliced
- ½ green bell pepper, halved and sliced
- 1 garlic clove, minced
- ½ teaspoon Himalayan salt
- ½ teaspoon black pepper, crushed
- ¼ teaspoon paprika
- 4 fresh sage leaves, thinly sliced
- 1 teaspoon oregano
- ¼ teaspoon red chili flakes
- 1 cup tempeh, crumbled
- 1 tablespoon parsley, chopped

Directions

1. Place sweet potato cubes in a medium pot over medium-high heat. Bring to a boil and let cook 5 minutes. Potatoes should be tender but not mushy. Drain and set aside.

2. Heat oil in a large skillet over medium-low heat. Add onion, both bell peppers, garlic and sweet potatoes. Cook 10 minutes, stirring frequently.

3. Stir in the salt, pepper, paprika, sage, oregano and chili flakes. Cook 2 minutes and then crumble in the tempeh. Cook another 2 minutes and then remove from heat.

4. Garnish with parsley before serving.

Papaya Breakfast Boat

Servings: 2

Total Time: 5 minutes

Ingredients

- 1 papaya, cut lengthwise in half and seeds removed
- 1 cup unsweetened yogurt
- 1 lime, zested
- 3 tablespoons raw oats
- 1 tablespoon unsweetened shredded coconut
- ½ banana, sliced
- ¼ cup raspberries
- 1 tablespoon walnuts, chopped
- 1 teaspoon chia seeds
- 1 teaspoon raw honey

Directions

1. Place papaya halves on plates and place yogurt on top of each.

2. Then top each half with lime zest, oats, coconut, banana, raspberries, walnuts, chia seeds.

3. Drizzle with honey and serve.

AM Quinoa Cookies

Servings: 2

Total Time: 25 minutes

Ingredients

- ¼ cup almond butter
- 1 tablespoon honey
- ½ medium ripe banana, mashed
- 1 egg, beaten
- ½ teaspoon vanilla
- ¼ teaspoon almond extract
- ¼ cup gluten-free oats
- ¼ cup quinoa flakes
- ½ teaspoon baking powder
- ¼ teaspoon Himalayan salt
- ¼ cup unsweetened, shredded coconut flakes, toasted
- 1 tablespoon chia seeds
- 1 teaspoon flaxseed, ground

Directions

1. Preheat oven to 350°F/180°C and line a baking tray with parchment paper.

2. In a large bowl, combine the almond butter, honey, banana, egg, vanilla and almond extract.

3. In a medium-sized bowl, combine the oats, quinoa flakes, baking powder, salt, coconut flakes, chia seeds and flaxseed.

4. Add the oat mixture to the almond butter mixture and stir well to combine.

5. Using 2 tablespoons as a guide, form small balls and place dough onto the baking tray until all dough is used.

6. Bake in the oven for 15 minutes.

7. Remove and let cool before serving.

Savory Breakfast Bowl

Servings: 1

Total Time: 20 minutes

Ingredients

- ½ cup rolled oats
- ½ cup unsweetened almond milk
- ½ cup water
- ¼ teaspoon Himalayan salt
- ¼ teaspoon black pepper, crushed
- 1 cup spinach
- 1 tablespoon nutritional yeast
- 1 teaspoon lemon zest
- ½ teaspoon turmeric
- ¼ teaspoon red chili flakes
- 1/3 cup lentils, cooked
- 1 tablespoon green onions, sliced

Directions

1. In a medium saucepan over medium heat, add oats, almond milk, water, salt and pepper. Bring to a boil and then reduce heat to low and simmer 5-10 minutes or until liquid is absorbed.

2. Stir in the spinach, nutritional yeast, lemon zest, turmeric, chili flakes and lentils.

3. Remove from heat and garnish with green onions before serving.

Almond Butter & Jelly Overnight Oats

Servings: 1

Total Time: 10 minutes plus 8 hours chill time

Ingredients

- ½ cup rolled oats
- ¾ cup unsweetened almond milk
- ½ teaspoon vanilla extract
- 1 teaspoon chia seeds
- 1 tablespoon almond butter
- 1 tablespoon sliced almonds
- 4 raspberries, sliced

Raspberry Jam

- ¼ cup raspberries, mashed
- 1 teaspoon honey
- 1 tablespoon chia seeds

Directions

1. In a small bowl, place the ¼ cup mashed raspberries, honey and 1 tablespoon chia seeds. Combine well and set aside in the fridge for 10 minutes.

2. Place oats, almond milk, vanilla, chia seeds and 1 tablespoon of raspberry mixture in a small jar and mix well. Cover and let sit in the fridge overnight.

3. In the morning, add almond butter, sliced almonds and remaining raspberries before serving.

Broccoli & Sprouts Savory Oats

Servings: 1

Total Time: 15 minutes

Ingredients

- 1 tablespoon olive oil
- 1 shallot, sliced
- 1 teaspoon nutritional yeast
- 1 teaspoon cayenne pepper
- ½ cup rolled oats
- ¾ cup unsweetened almond milk
- ¼ cup water
- 1 cup broccoli florets, steamed and chopped small
- ½ teaspoon Himalayan salt
- ½ teaspoon black pepper, crushed
- ½ cup alfalfa sprouts

Directions

1. In a medium saucepan over medium heat add the oil, shallot, yeast and cayenne pepper. Cook 5 minutes and then add the oats, almond milk and water.

2. Bring to a boil and reduce heat to low. Cook 5 minutes until liquid is absorbed.

3. Stir in the broccoli, salt and pepper.

4. Remove from heat and top with sprouts before serving

Fruit & Millet Breakfast

Servings: 2

Total Time: 30 minutes

Ingredients

- ½ cup millet
- 1 cup water
- 2 tablespoons raisins
- 1 tablespoon currants
- ⅛ teaspoon cinnamon
- ⅛ teaspoon vanilla extract
- 1 cup unsweetened coconut milk, divided
- 1 teaspoon honey
- ½ cup raspberries
- ½ cup blueberries
- 1 teaspoon hemp hearts
- 1 teaspoon chia seeds
- 1 teaspoon mint, chopped

Directions

1. Place millet and water in a medium saucepan over medium heat. Bring to a boil and then add the raisins, currants, cinnamon and vanilla. Cover with a lid, reduce heat to low and let cook for another 10 minutes until liquid is absorbed.

2. Turn heat off and let sit for 10 minutes

3. Add coconut milk, honey, raspberries, blueberries, hemp hearts and chia seeds. Turn heat to low and let cook for 2 minutes.

4. Transfer to bowls and garnish with mint.

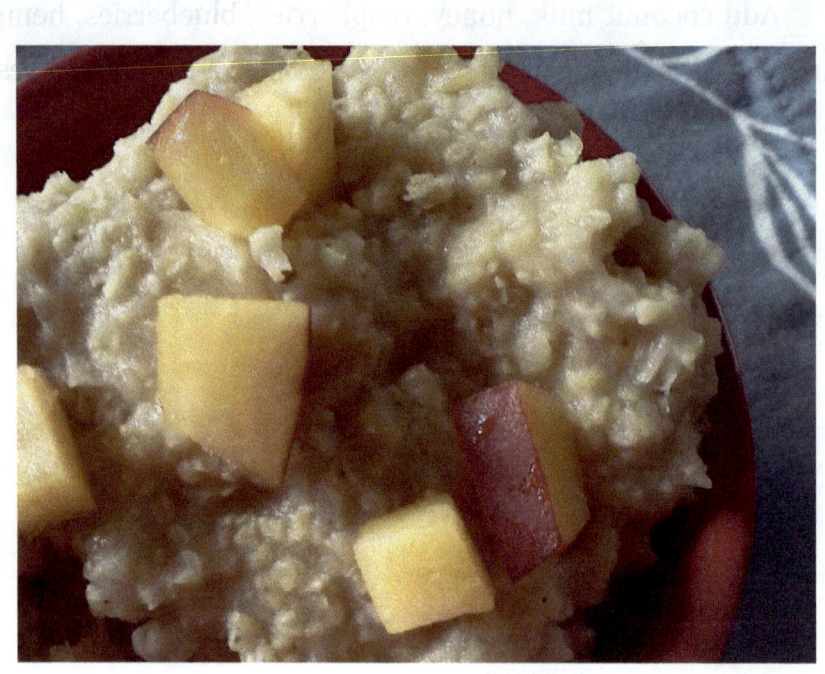

Avocado Breakfast Soup

Servings: 1

Total Time: 5 minutes

Ingredients

- 1 avocado
- 1 lime, zested and juiced
- ½ cup cucumber, roughly chopped
- ½ cup spinach
- 18 fresh mint leaves
- ⅛ teaspoon Himalayan salt
- 2 tablespoons coconut oil, melted
- 1 tablespoon pepitas
- 1 tablespoon green raisins

Directions

1. Place all the ingredients, except the pepitas and raisins in a food processor or blender and combine until smooth.
2. Transfer to a bowl and top with pepitas and green raisins.

Sweet Orange Oats

Servings: 2

Total Time: 12 minutes

Ingredients

- 1 cup sweet potato, cubed, roasted and mashed
- ½ cup oats
- 1/3 cup carrots, grated
- 1 cup unsweetened almond milk
- 2 tablespoons orange juice
- ½ teaspoon ground cinnamon
- ½ teaspoon nutmeg
- ¼ teaspoon Himalayan salt
- 1 teaspoon chia seeds
- ½ persimmon, sliced
- 1 tablespoon orange zest

Directions

1. In a medium saucepan over medium-low heat, combine mashed sweet potato, oats, carrots, almond milk, orange juice, cinnamon, nutmeg and salt.

2. Bring to a low boil, reduce heat to low and simmer until liquid is absorbed.

3. Stir in chia seeds and garnish with persimmon slices and orange zest to serve.

Greek Zucchini Cups

Servings: 2

Total Time: 10 minutes

Ingredients

- 2 medium zucchinis, cut into 2 inch pieces and each piece slightly cored to form a cup
- 1 cucumber, finely grated
- 1 cup plain Greek yogurt
- 1 garlic clove, minced
- 1 tablespoon dill, chopped
- 1 tablespoon parsley, chopped
- 1 tablespoon lemon juice
- ½ teaspoon Himalayan salt
- ½ teaspoon black pepper, crushed
- 10 black olives, finely chopped
- 2 tablespoons sprouts

Directions

1. Prepare zucchini cups and set aside.

2. In a bowl, mix together cucumber, yogurt, garlic, dill, parsley, lemon juice, salt and pepper. Spoon into zucchini cups.

3. Top each cup with some of the olives and sprouts.

Endive & Watercress Boats

Servings: 2

Total Time: 5 minutes

Ingredients

- 3 cups fresh spinach
- 1 avocado
- 1/2 cup parsley
- ¼ cup mint
- 1 tablespoon lemon juice
- 1 garlic clove
- 1 teaspoon Himalayan salt
- 10 endive leaves
- 1 cup watercress

Directions

1. Add all ingredients except the endive leaves & watercress to a blender or food processor and blend until smooth, this will form the dip.

2. Scoop dip into each of the endive leaves and top with watercress.

Toasted Trail Mix

Servings: 2

Total Time: 5 minutes

Ingredients

- 3 tablespoons coconut chips, toasted
- 3 tablespoons walnuts, toasted
- 2 tablespoons almonds, toasted
- 2 tablespoons raisins
- 1 tablespoon pepitas, toasted
- Pinch Himalayan salt

Directions

1. Combine all ingredients and divide into two equal portions

Chickpea Avocado Cups

Servings: 1

Total Time: 5 minutes

Ingredients

- 1 very ripe avocado
- ½ cup cooked chickpeas
- ½ tomato, diced
- 1 shallot, diced
- 2 tablespoons olive oil
- 1 tablespoon lemon juice
- ½ teaspoon Himalayan salt
- ½ teaspoon black pepper, crushed
- 1 tablespoon fresh basil, chopped
- 1 teaspoon oregano

Directions

1. In a small bowl combine chickpeas, tomato, shallot, olive oil, lemon juice, salt and black pepper. Set aside and let rest 5 minutes.

2. Slice the avocado in half lengthwise and remove the pit. Spoon the chickpea and tomato mixture over the middle of each avocado.

3. Garnish with oregano and fresh basil.

Spicy Cocoa-Coco Truffles

Servings: 2

Total Time: 10 minutes

Ingredients

- 2 cups pitted dates
- ½ cup almond meal
- 1/3 cup shredded unsweetened coconut
- 6 tablespoons raw cacao (or unsweetened cocoa) powder, divided
- ¼ teaspoon sea salt
- ¼ teaspoon cayenne pepper

Directions

1. Using a food processor on the pulse setting combine the dates, almond meal and shredded coconut until crumbly.

2. Add in 3 tablespoons of the cacao, the sea salt and the cayenne. Blend until the mixture becomes a sticky paste and begins to form a ball.

3.	Tear off pieces of the dough and shape into 6 balls. Place remaining cacao on a plate and roll each ball lightly in the cacao.

Adult Ants on a Log

Servings: 1

Total Time: 5 minutes

Ingredients

- 3 celery stalks, trimmed
- 3 tablespoons almond butter
- 1 tablespoon raisins
- 1 teaspoon sunflower seeds

Directions

1. Spread almond butter evenly on the celery stalks.
2. Top each piece of celery with raisins and sunflower seeds.

Asian Cucumber Slaw

Servings: 1

Total Time: 15 minutes

Ingredients

- 1 large cucumber, diced
- 1 garlic clove, minced
- 1 teaspoon fresh ginger, grated
- 2 tablespoons toasted sesame seed oil
- 1 tablespoon brown rice vinegar
- ¼ teaspoon Himalayan salt
- ¼ teaspoon black pepper, crushed
- 1 tablespoon cilantro, chopped

Directions

1. In a medium bowl, whisk together garlic, ginger, sesame seed oil, vinegar, salt and pepper.
2. Add cucumber and cilantro. Let sit for 5 minutes before serving.

Broiled Grapefruit

Servings: 1

Total Time: 5 minutes

Ingredients

- ¼ grapefruit
- 1 teaspoon raw honey
- 1 teaspoon almond, crushed
- Pinch flaked sea salt

Directions

1. Place grapefruit on a broiler pan and broil on high for 3-5 minutes or until lightly brûléed.

2. Spread raw honey on top of the grapefruit and sprinkle with almonds and flaked sea salt.

Coconut Curry Soup

Servings: 2

Total Time: 5 minutes

Ingredients

- 1 ½ teaspoons coconut oil
- 1 inch piece of ginger, grated
- 2 garlic cloves, minced
- 1 lime, zested
- 1 teaspoon ground coriander
- 1 teaspoon cumin
- ½ teaspoon turmeric
- ½ teaspoon ground mustard
- ½ teaspoon red chili flakes
- ½ teaspoon Himalayan salt
- ¼ teaspoon black pepper, crushed
- 2 small sweet potatoes, peeled and cut into 1 inch pieces
- 1 15 ounce can of full fat coconut milk
- 1 cup filtered water

- ¼ cup cilantro, chopped
- 1 tablespoon pumpkin seeds, toasted
- 2 tablespoons green onions, sliced

Directions

1. In a large pot over medium heat place coconut oil, ginger, garlic and lime zest. Cook for 5 minutes or until fragrant, being sure to stir frequently.

2. Add coriander, cumin, turmeric, mustard and chili flakes. Continue to stir for another minute before adding in coconut milk, sweet potatoes and water. Bring to a boil then lower heat and simmer for 1 hour.

3. After an hour, turn heat off and let cool completely before adding to a food processor or blender and pureeing until smooth.

4. Place mixture back in the pot and bring to a simmer. Season with salt and pepper.

5. Pour mixture into bowls and garnish with cilantro, pumpkin seeds and green onions.

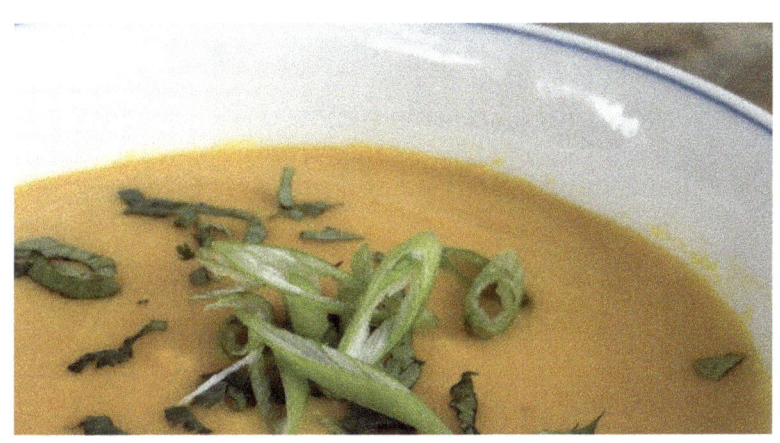

Chilled Avocado Cilantro Soup

Servings: 2

Total Time: 5 minutes plus 30 minutes chill time

Ingredients

- 2 cups water
- 1 cup spinach
- 1 avocado, pitted and skin removed
- 1 small cucumber, peeled and seeds removed
- ½ cup cilantro, chopped
- 1 lemon, zested and juiced
- 1 teaspoon Himalayan salt
- ½ teaspoon black pepper, crushed
- ¼ teaspoon cayenne pepper
- 1 inch piece ginger, grated
- 1 garlic clove, grated
- 1 tablespoon cilantro, finely chopped
- 2 tablespoons cucumber, finely diced

Directions

1. Place all ingredients except for the cilantro and cucumber in a blender and process until smooth to create the soup. Add water if the mixture is too thick.

2. Chill the soup for 30 minutes before garnishing with remaining cilantro and cucumber.

Cooling Cucumber Slice Snack

Servings: 2

Total Time: 5 minutes plus 15 minutes chill time

Ingredients

- 1 large cucumber, sliced
- 2 garlic cloves, grated
- 1 tablespoon green onion, sliced
- 1 tablespoon toasted sesame oil
- 2 teaspoons apple cider vinegar
- ¼ teaspoon red chili flakes
- ⅛ teaspoon Himalayan salt
- ⅛ teaspoon black pepper, crushed
- 1 teaspoon black sesame seeds

Directions

1. In a medium bowl whisk together the garlic, green onion, sesame oil, vinegar, chili flakes, salt and pepper.

2. Toss in the cucumber and let sit in the fridge for 15 minutes before sprinkling with sesame seeds and serving.

Spicy Tortilla Soup

Servings: 2

Total Time: 20 minutes

Ingredients

- 1 tablespoon olive oil
- 1 shallot, diced
- 1 jalapeno, seeded and diced small
- 1 red bell pepper, diced
- 1 tomato, diced
- 1 teaspoon cumin
- 1 teaspoon cayenne pepper
- 1 teaspoon red chili flakes
- 1 cup water
- 1 cup vegetable broth
- ½ cup cilantro, chopped
- 1 cup spinach, chopped
- 1 lime, zested and juiced
- ¼ teaspoon Himalayan salt

- ¼ teaspoon black pepper, crushed
- 1 sprouted tortilla wrap, cut into strips and toasted
- 1 ripe avocado, diced

Directions

1. In a large pot heat olive oil over medium low heat and add shallot, jalapeno, red bell pepper and tomato for 5 minutes. Add cumin, cayenne and chili flakes and stir for one minute before adding water and vegetable broth.

2. Bring to a boil and then reduce heat and simmer for 15 minutes.

3. Reduce heat and stir in spinach, cilantro, lime zest, lime juice, salt and pepper.

4. Place in bowls and garnish with tortilla strips and avocado.

Raw Green Gazpacho

Servings: 2

Total Time: 5 minutes plus 2 hours chill time

Ingredients

- 1 medium tomatoes
- 1 green bell pepper, seeds removed and chopped
- 1 tablespoon olive oil
- 1 cup parsley, chopped
- ½ cup cilantro, chopped
- ½ jalapeno, seeded and chopped
- 1 lemon, juiced
- 1 avocado, pitted and flesh removed
- 1 cup vegetable broth
- 1 cup water
- ½ cucumber, diced
- 1 shallot, diced
- 1 tablespoon cilantro, finely chopped
- ½ teaspoon paprika

- ½ teaspoon cumin
- ½ teaspoon cayenne pepper
- ¼ teaspoon Himalayan salt
- ¼ teaspoon black pepper, crushed
- 2 tablespoons green onions

Directions

1. Add all ingredients except the green onions to a blender and mix until well combined.

2. Chill for 2 hours before garnishing with green onions to serve.

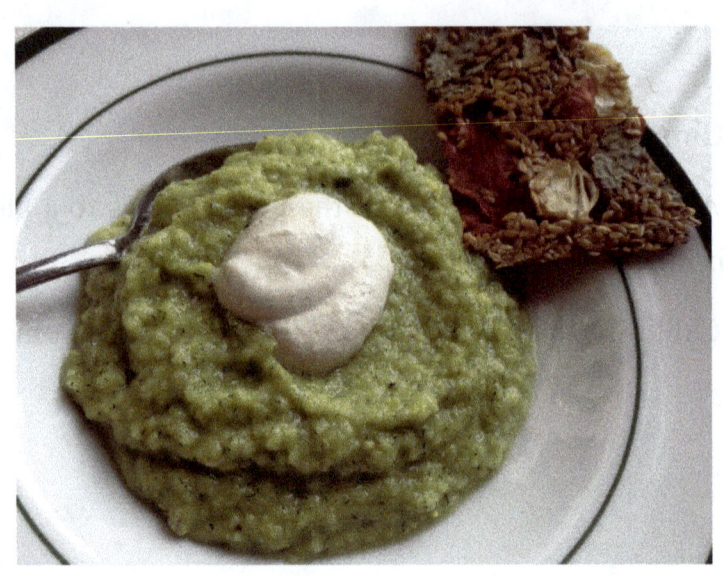

www.ingramcontent.com/pod-product-compliance
Lightning Source LLC
Chambersburg PA
CBHW070733030426
42336CB00013B/1959